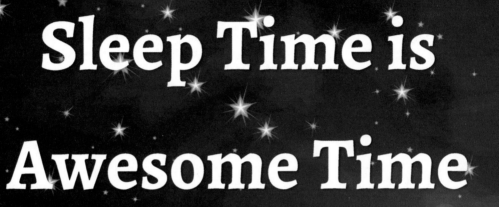

Sleep Time is Awesome Time

CHARLES C. MARTIN

www.haharain.com / www.charlesCmartin.com
Story written and arranged by Charles C. Martin. Special thanks to cover art by Aeoroartist and graphic artists; Andrey Alyukhin, Andrei Krauchuk, Viktoriia Kryzhanovska, Lukas Gojda, Irina Akhremenko, Corey Ford, Pedro Angeles-Flores, Robert Davies, Norbert Buchholz, Вадим Ерофеев, Алексей Овчинников, Viacheslav Votchitsev, Viacheslav Votchitsev, Liane Matrisch, Martin Valigursky, Antony Laurent, Luca Oleastri, Nataliia Natykach, Philip Morley, Anton Kalinichenko, Anna Anisimova, Stephanie Frey, Avesh Kumar, Elin Marianne Podsedník, Bogdan Zagan, Laurent Renault, Vitezslav Valka, Ebru Erdogan, Ksenia Samorukova, Valerii Egorov, James Steidl, Olga Yakovenko, sawitree kromkrathog)Эрфан Нуриев, Sabri deniz KIZIL, Quentin Rutsaert, Volodymy Grinko, Raman Maisei, Stephan Marques, Andrey Kuzmin, Ratchapon Yanyongdecha, Matthew Cole, Ann Triling, Oleksandr Lupol, Michael Flippo, Elena Semenko, Okan Başoğlu, Viktoriia Dobrianska, Anna Stsonn, Maxim Borovkov.

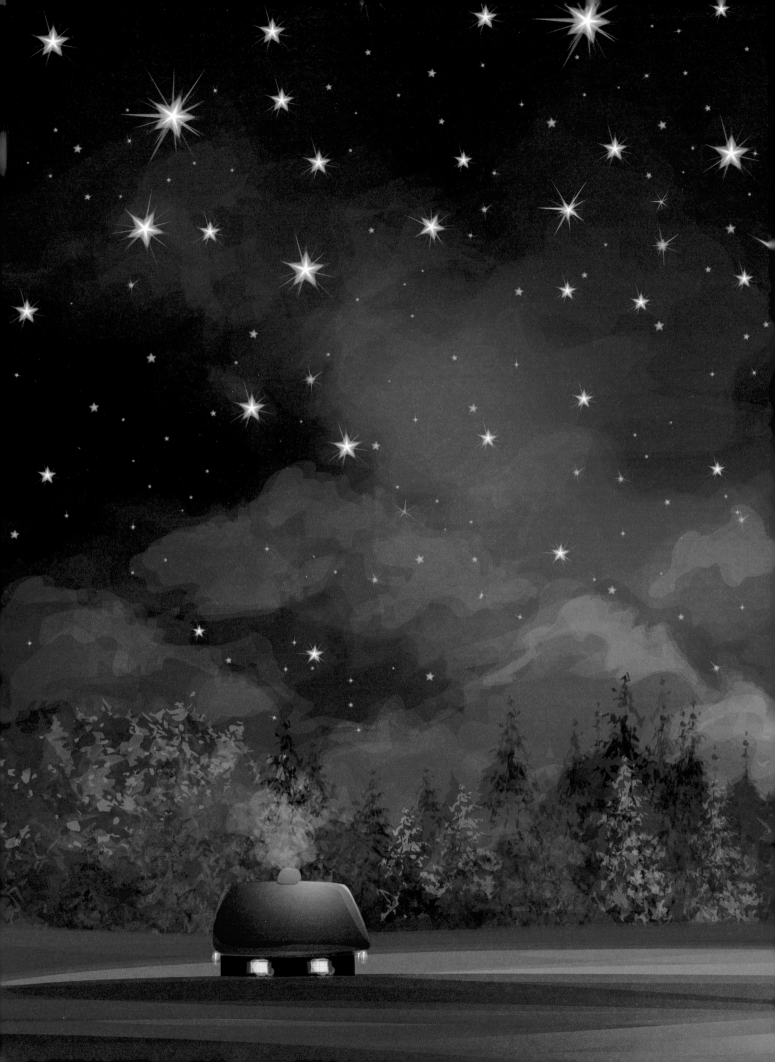

Congratulations!

You get to go to SLEEP!

Sleep time is

Awesome

time

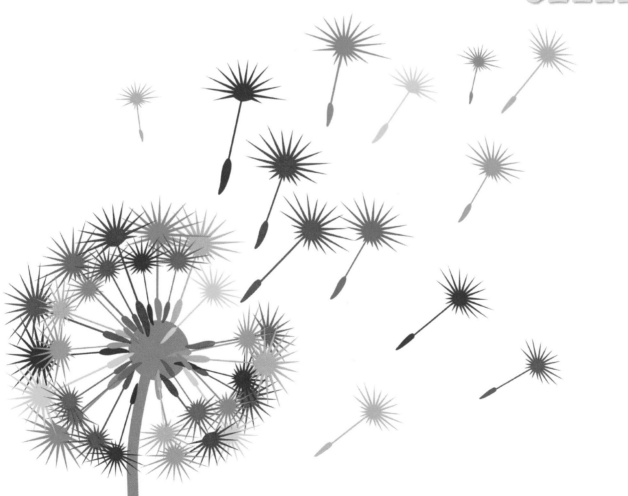

Sleep time is YOUR time. That's right, it's just for YOU.

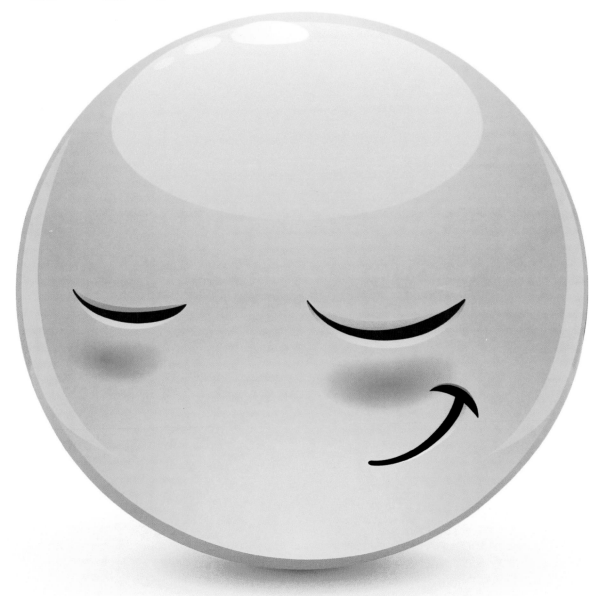

Now that you are comfy, cozy, and in bed, do you know what that means?

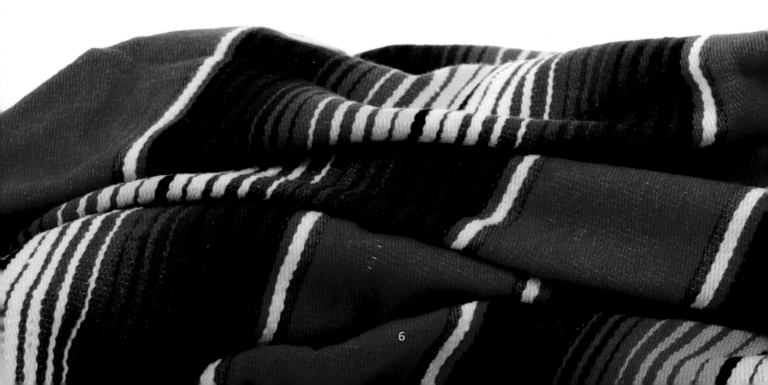

NO
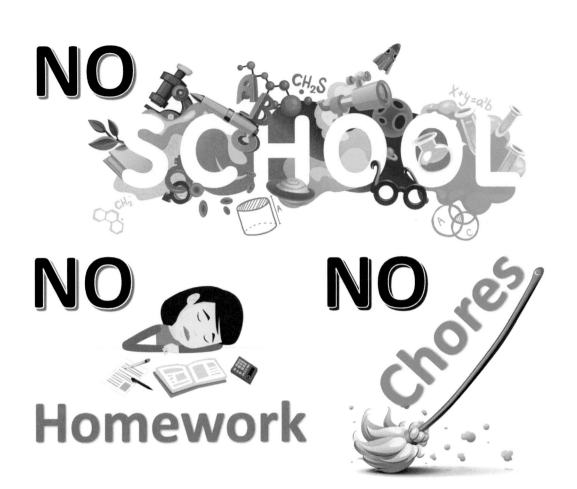
SCHOOL

NO
Homework

NO
chores

You are FREE to CHILL and CHARGE.

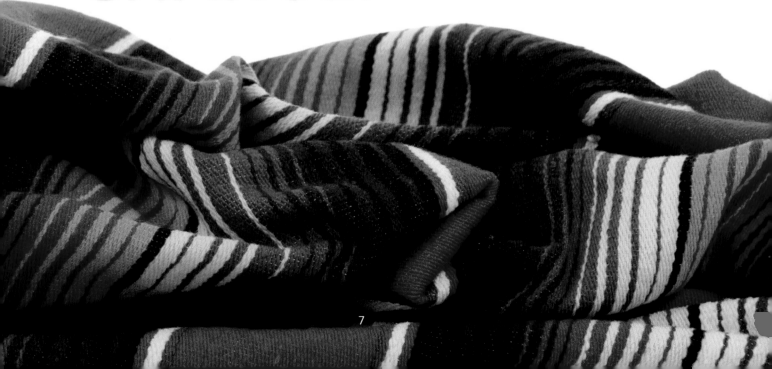

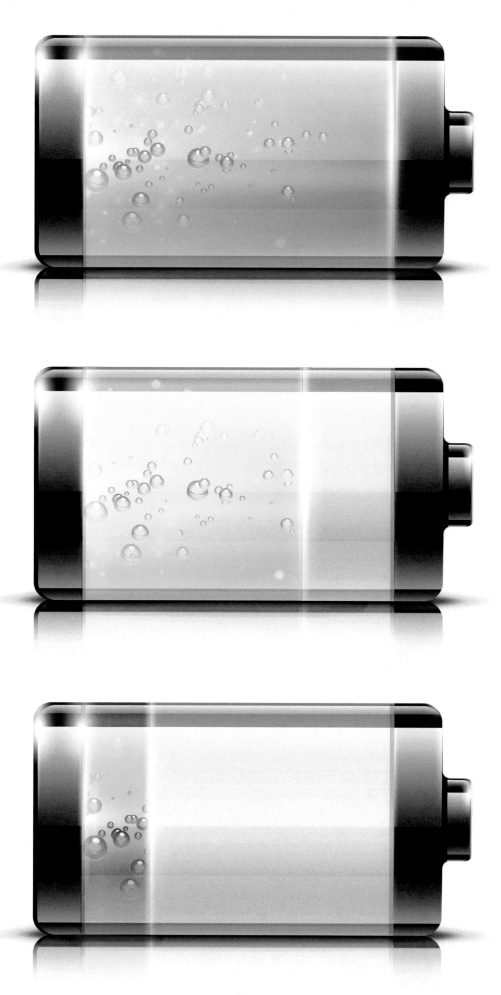

YES!

Just like a phone needs

to be **charged**,

so do you!

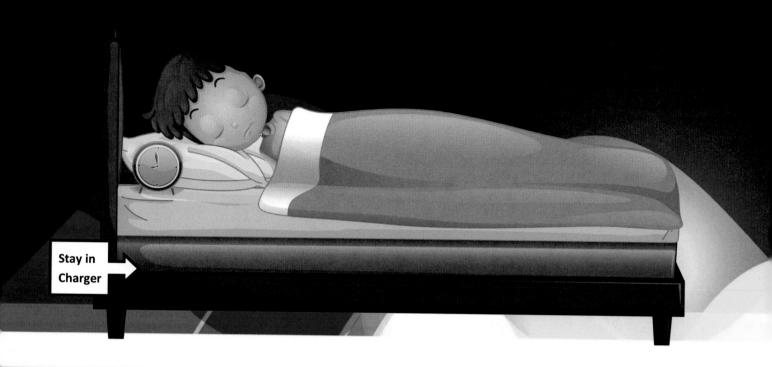

Stay in Charger

Your bed is the charger, so make sure to

stay in it!

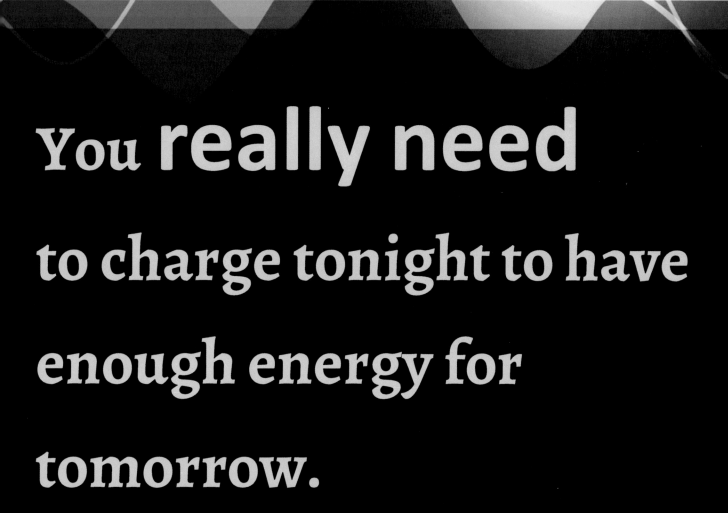

You **really need** to charge tonight to have enough energy for tomorrow.

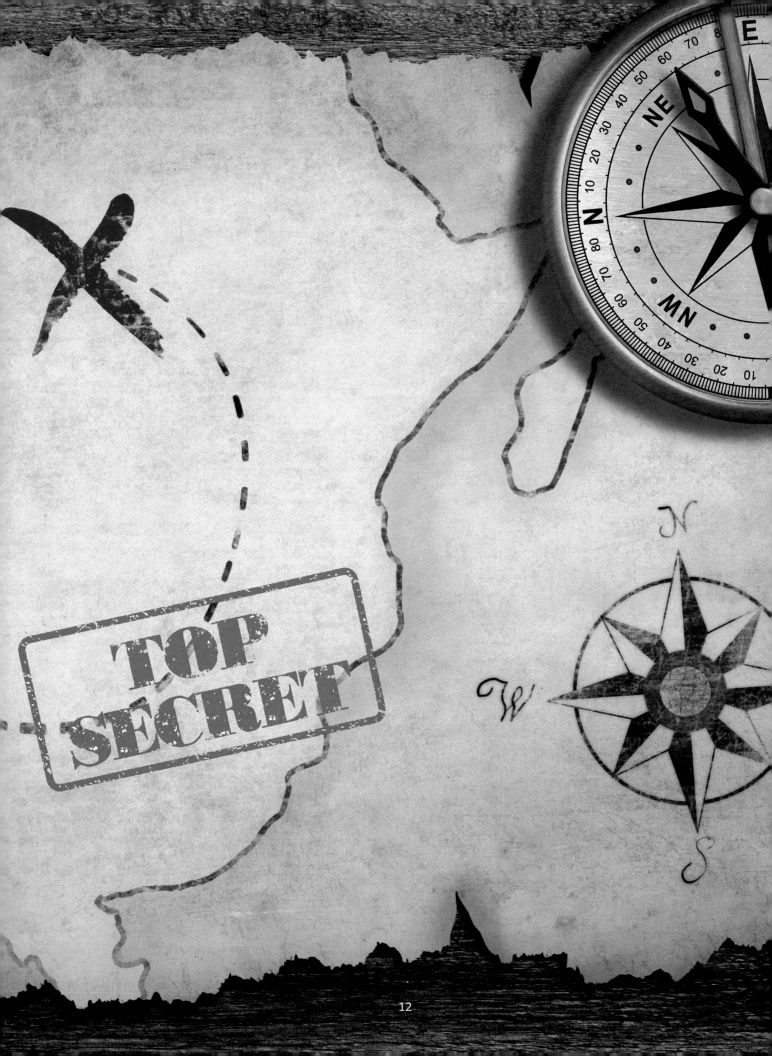

TOP SECRET

Now, I'm going to tell you a very, very important secret. You have one amazing, built-in tool to help you go to sleep. Do you know what it is?

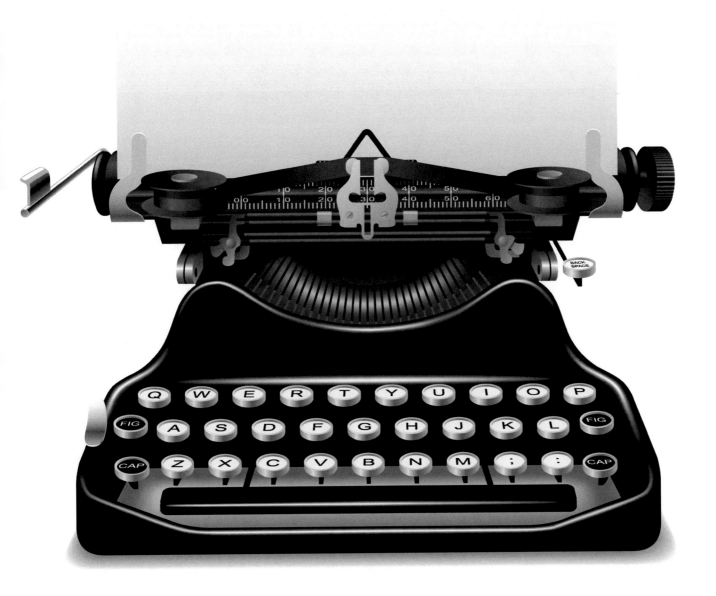

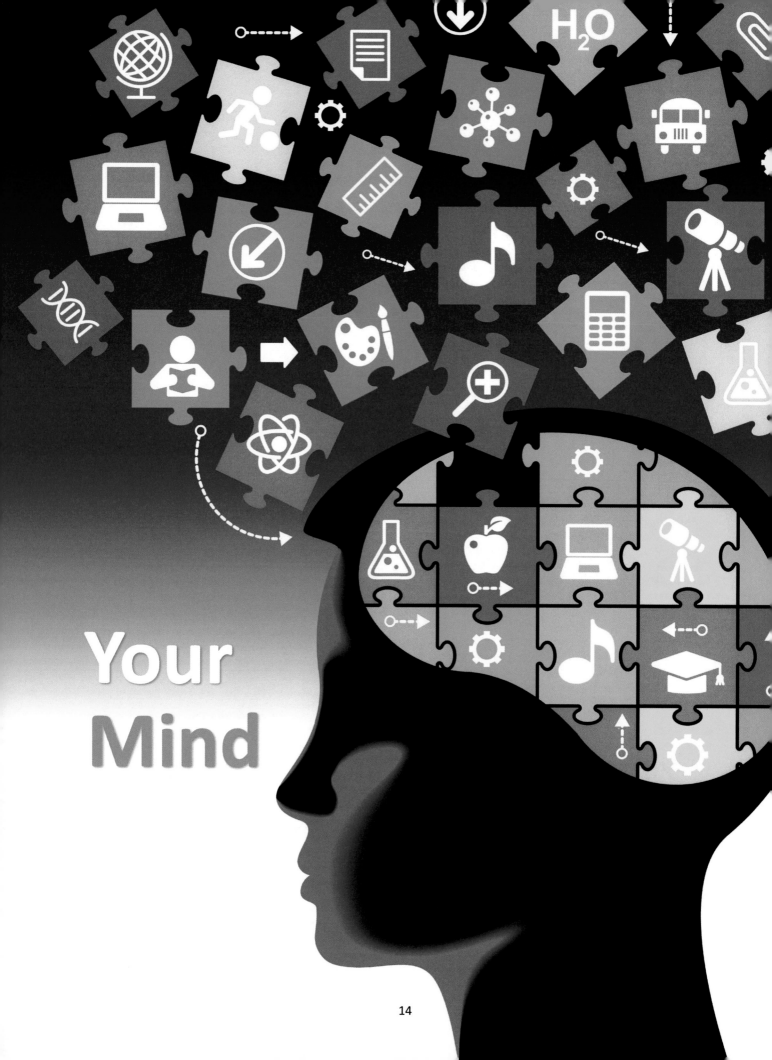

Your
Mind

Your mind is a **big,**

beautiful,

wonderful,

creation. It is also **very**

powerful.

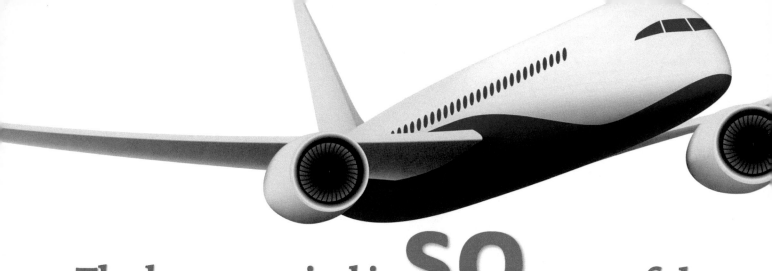

The human mind is **SO** powerful it has been used to create airplanes, pyramids, computers, electricity, and even spaceships.

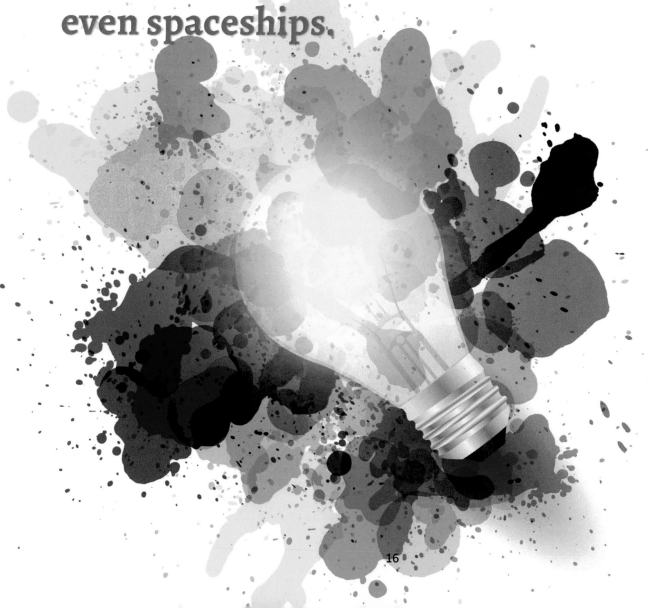

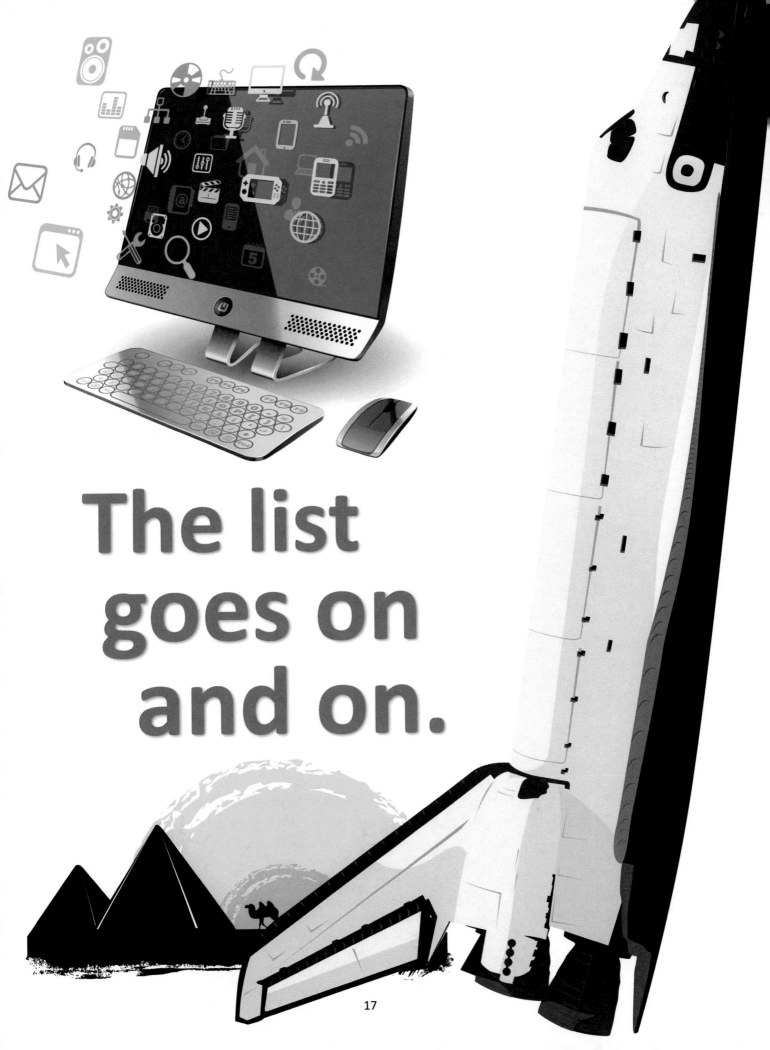

The list goes on and on.

Wow! That's a **WHOLE LOTTA** power you have in that head of yours.

You can even use it
to help you sleep, but
there's a **CATCH**.
It can also keep you
up at night.

So, here's the

secret.

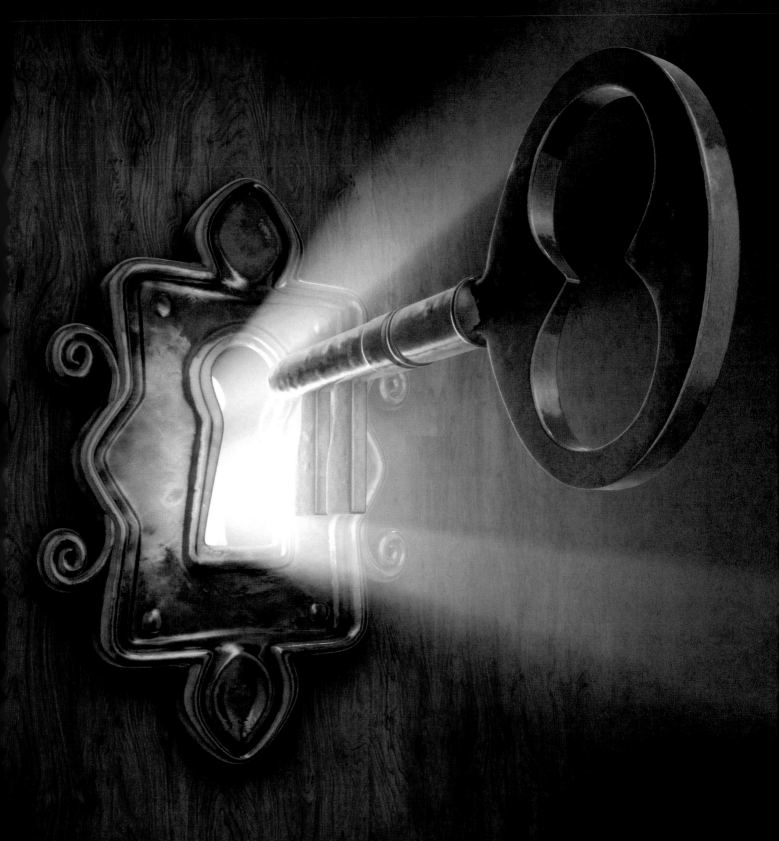

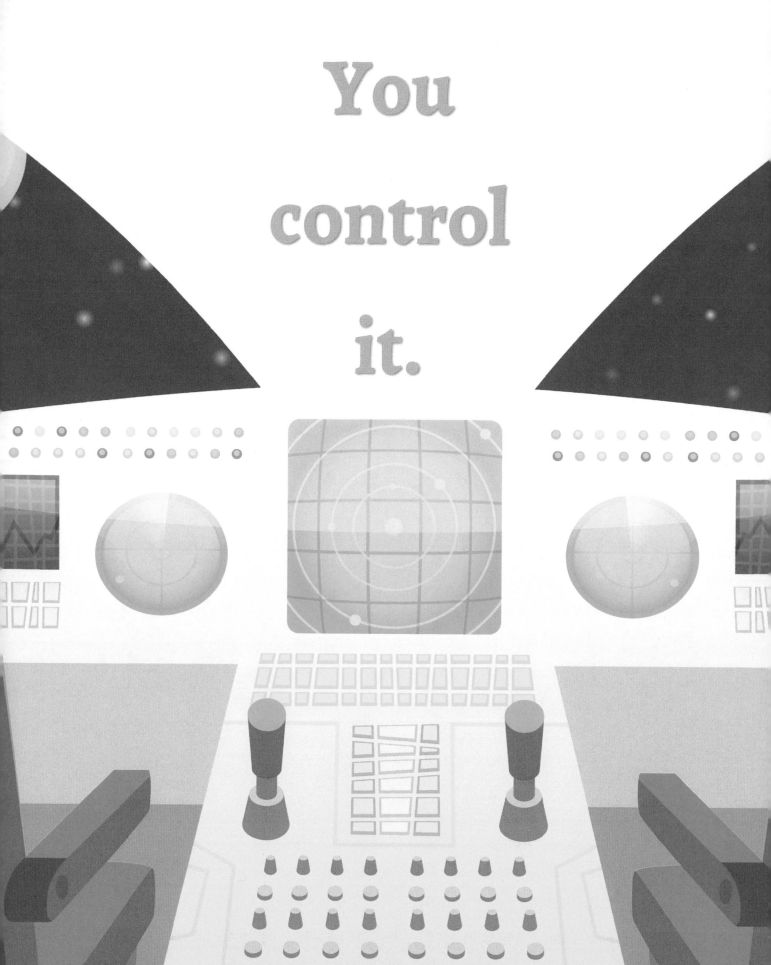

It's

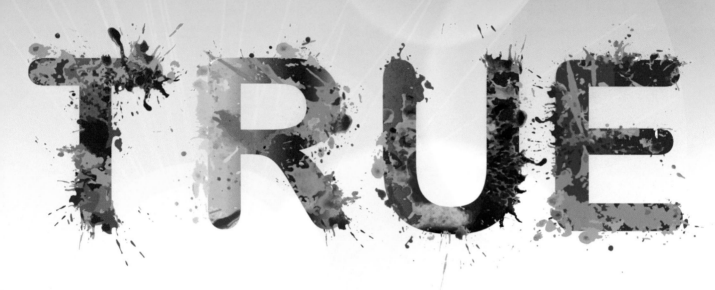

TRUE

Don't believe me?

Okay, check

this out.

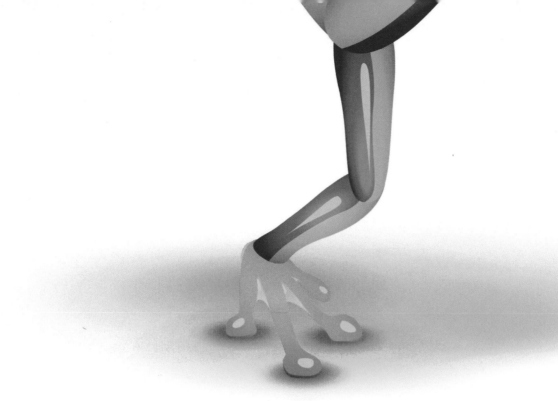

On the count of **3**, say an animal, any animal. **Ready? 1,2,3.**

Now **imagine** the animal dancing.

Got it? Keep imagining. Dance, baby dance, oh yeah! Great, now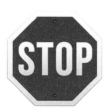

This time on the count of **3** think of a place, any place, and say it out loud.

1,2,3. Now **imagine** yourself flying through that place. No plane, no helicopter,

YOU CAN FLY.

Got it? Keep flying.... Keep flying...

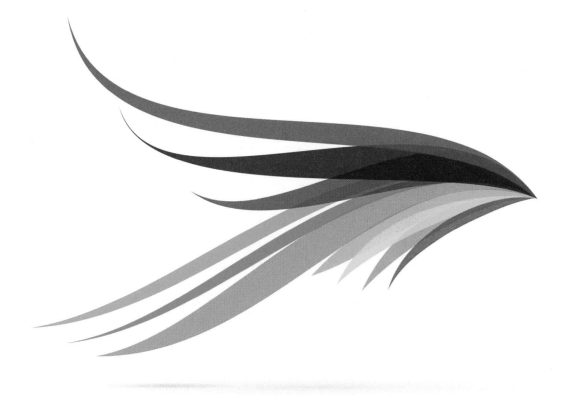

SEE!

Your mind is YOURS. You can stop and start thoughts just like a video game, and the more you practice, the better you will get.

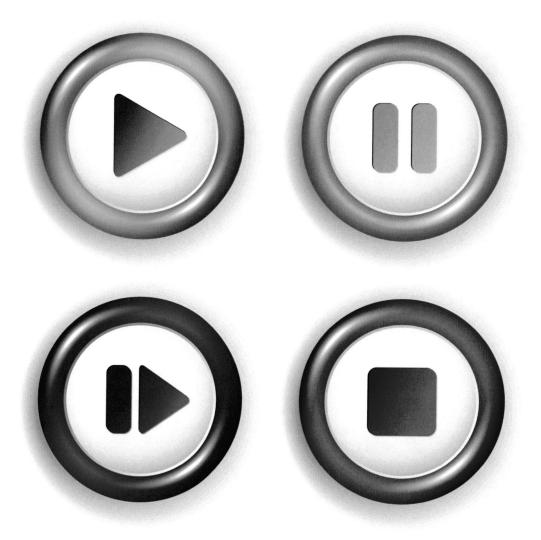

Remember, **you** have the controls.

Now sometimes you may find that you let go of the controls and are thinking about something weird and scary, like this dude.

STOP that thought, **DITCH** that loser, and put your mind on what you want.

You're the BOSS.

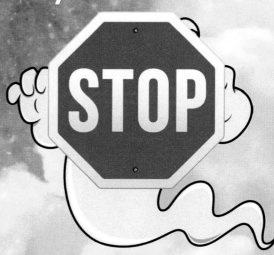

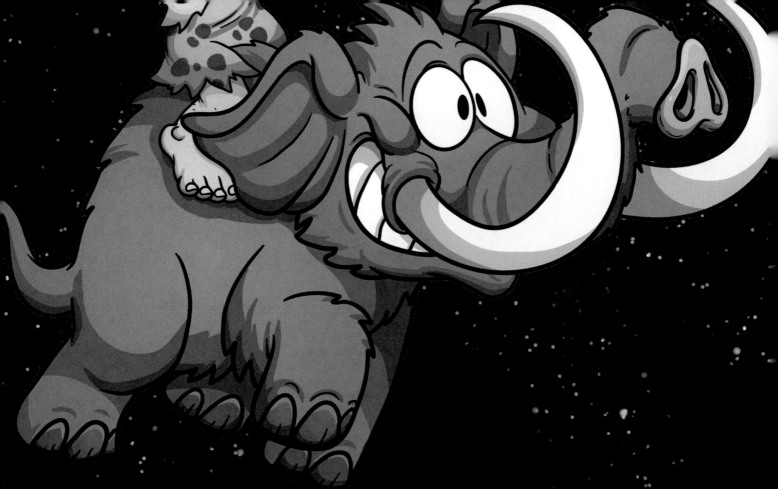

You've got this!

Now when you first close your eyes, you may choose to **imagine** fun thoughts filled with exciting adventures.

COOL!

After a little while you may want to switch to calm thoughts that will help you go to sleep.

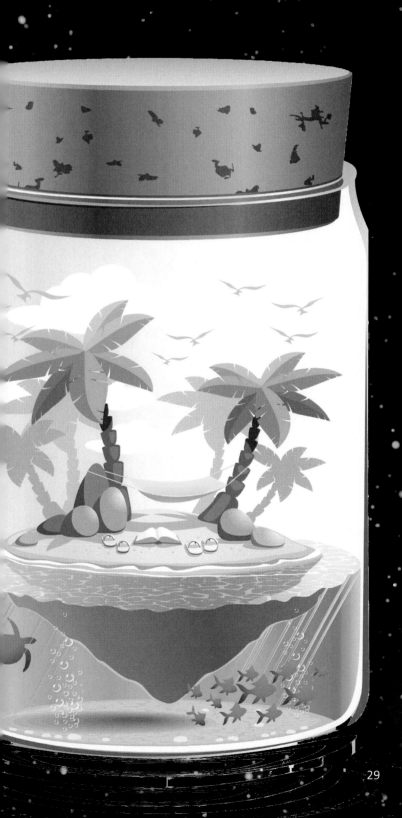

So, let's throw out some **ideas!** I get to go first. Alright,

I SHALL START WITH fun thoughts. Get ready to have your awesome mind **blown.**

Fun thought idea #1

Okay, so, you live across the river

in a cupcake palace!

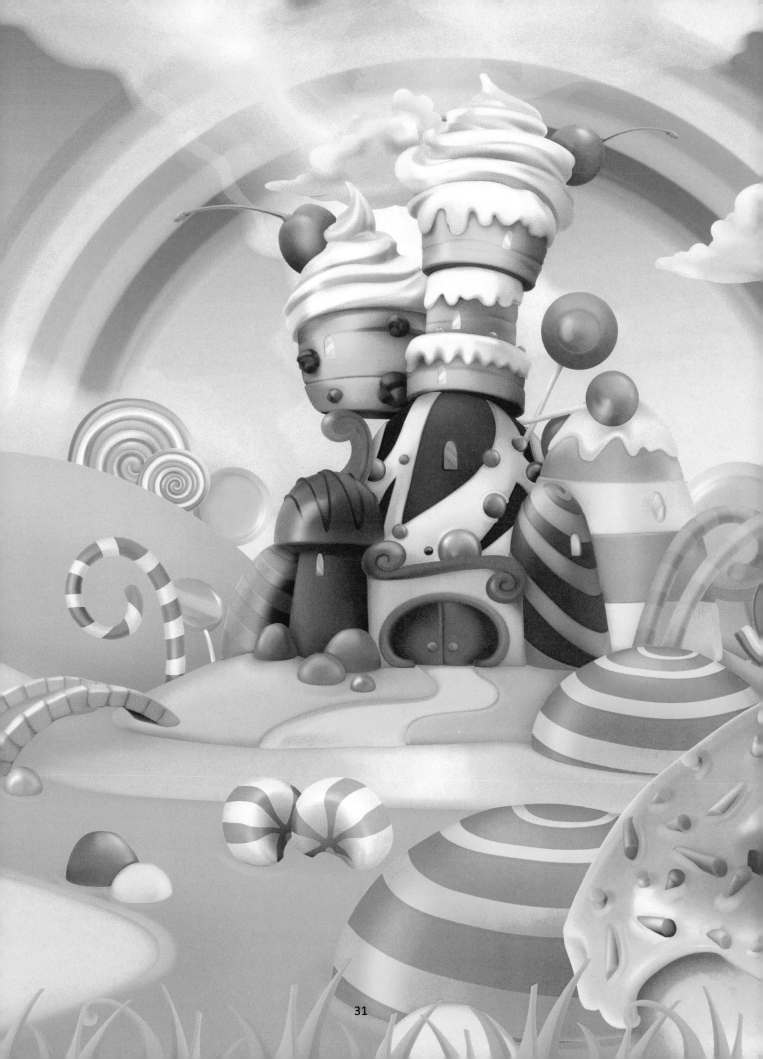

Fun thought idea #2

You have a beautiful pet elephant that you ride to school every morning!

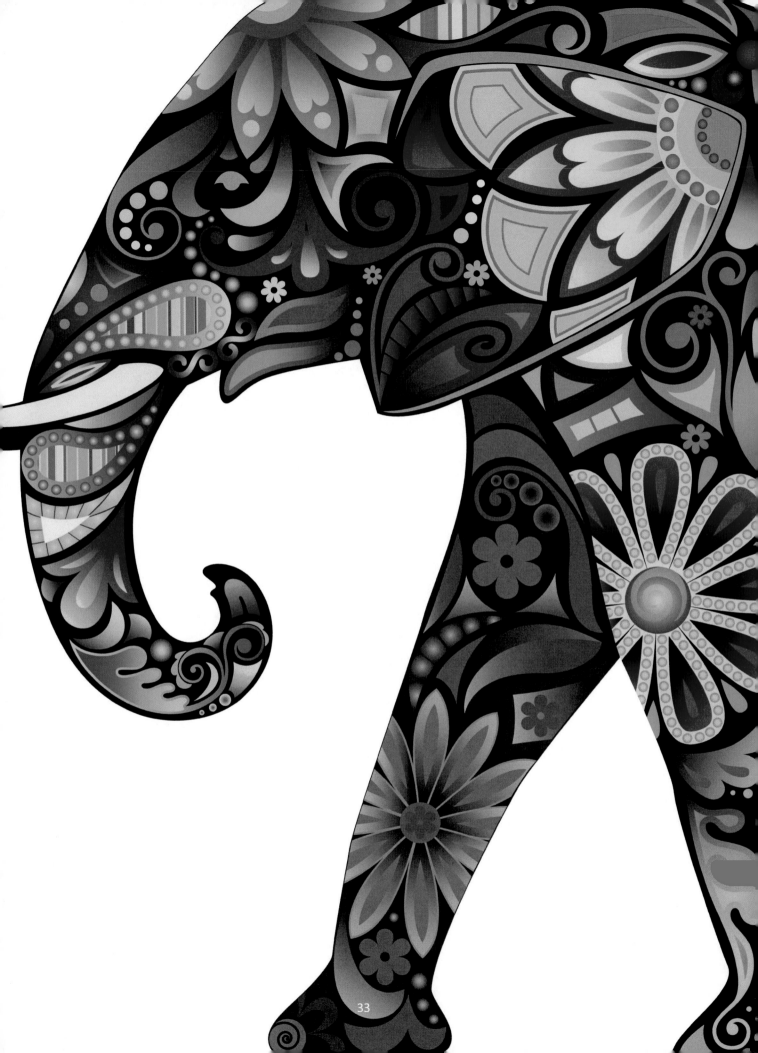

33

Fun thought idea #3

You are captain of the Galacticore Battleship and patrol galaxies 1,000 light years away!

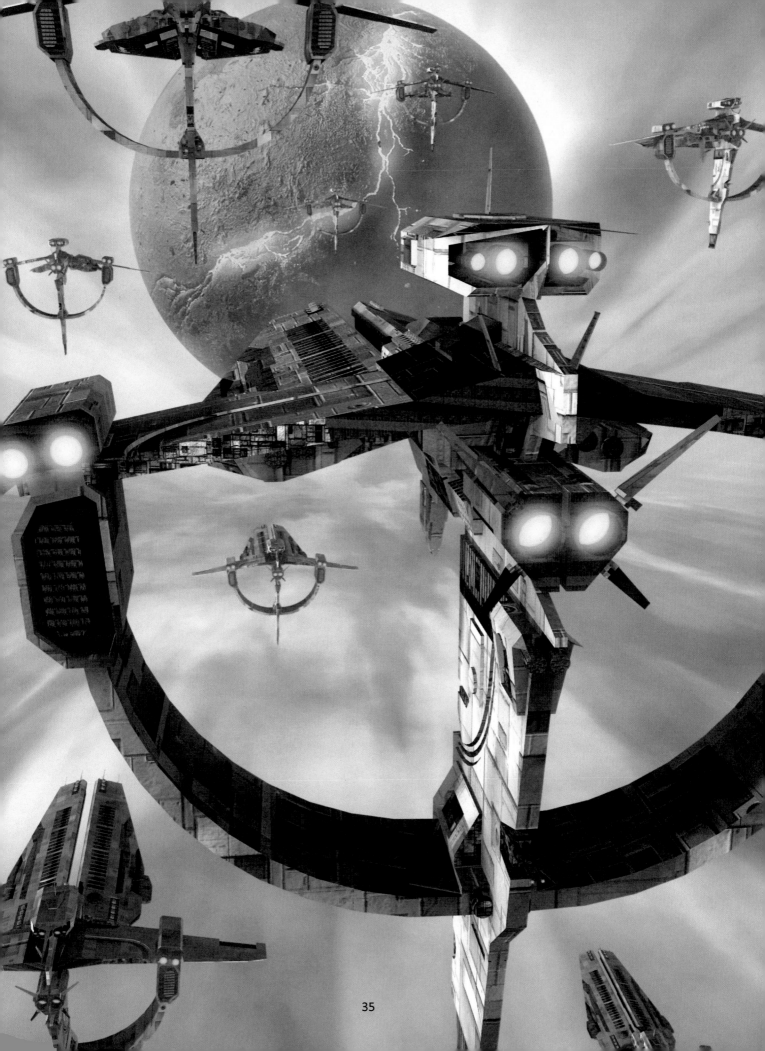

Okay, now for some
calm thoughts.

Calm thought idea #1

It's snowing outside your cabin and you
are asleep on a cozy couch in front of a
warm fireplace.

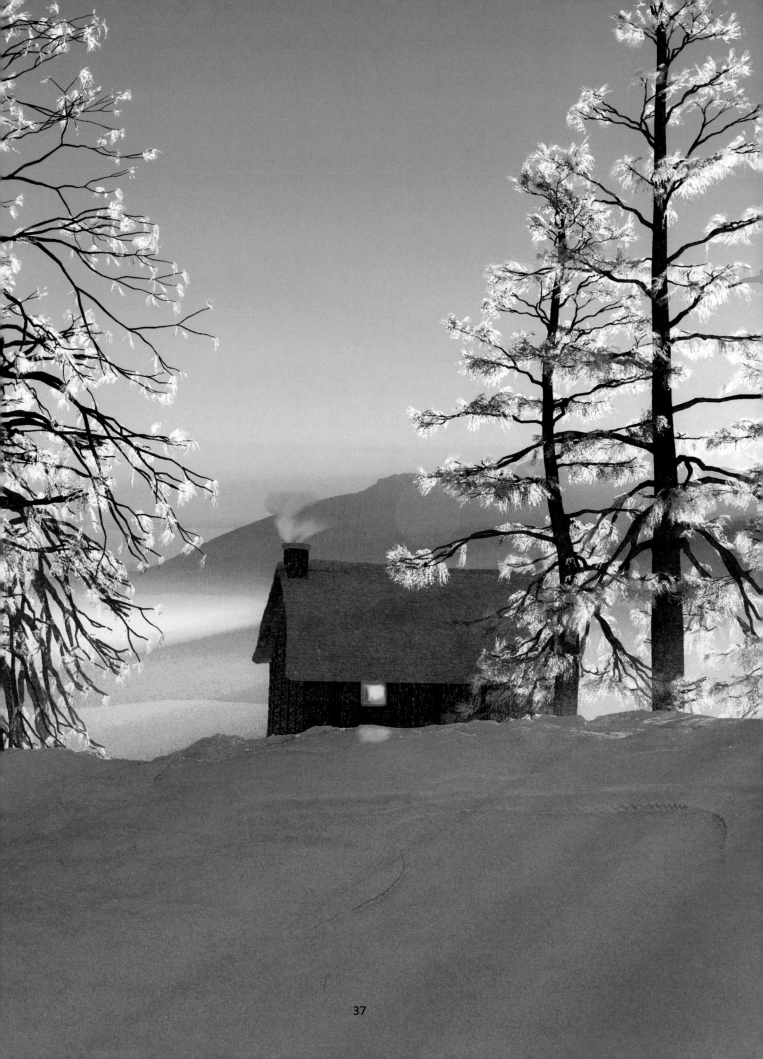

Calm thought idea #2

You're listening to the sound of waves while you fall asleep in a hammock on a beautiful beach.

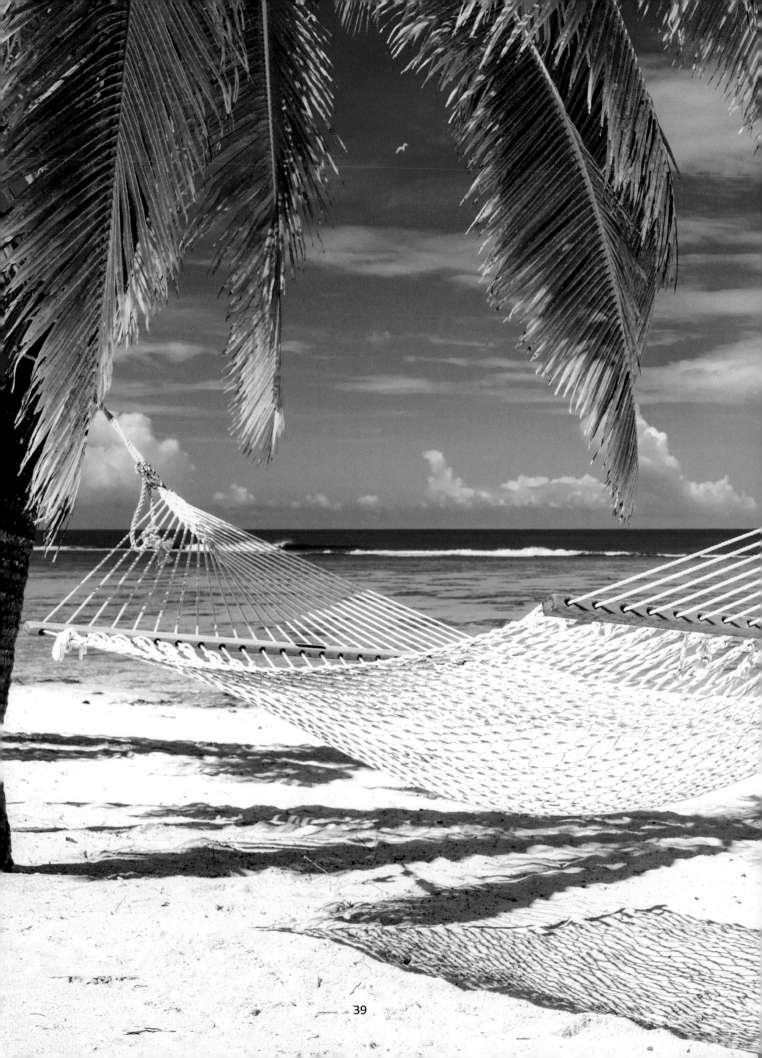

Calm thought idea #3

You are a chicken in a field. Wait....
scratch this one. Nobody wants to be a
chicken.

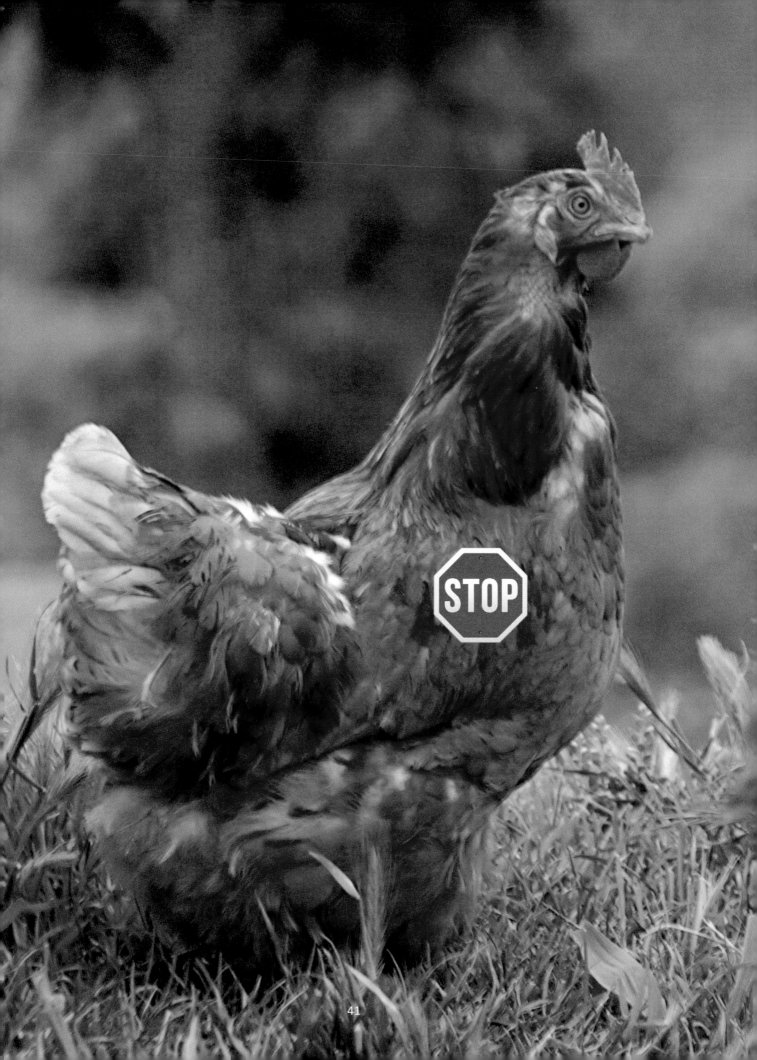

Okay, these are just silly pictures.

But YOUR mind is **powerful**
and **limitless.**
You know what?

I bet you have **MUCH** better ideas than me. So, I'm going to leave **you** with a few extra pages to write down some of your own.

Go for it!

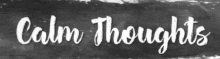

Calm Thoughts

Remember, sleep time is one of life's greatest gifts.

Enjoy it!

The End!